30 Winning Weight Loss Ways

Simple, easy, step-by-step expert diet guidance

By
Dr Phil Harley

ISBN-13: 978-1530543229

ISBN-10: 1530543223

"People often say that motivation doesn't last. Well, neither does bathing - that's why we recommend it daily."

Zig Ziglar.

Money Back Guarantee

*I do not know you or your life situation. But what I do know is that these winning ways work for thousands of my patients. My guarantee is that if you follow the steps in here, the thirty action plans, you **will** see results. I guarantee if you keep up these actions that the results will stay. If you follow these steps life long, you will reap the benefits life long. If you do not succeed, simply let me know and I will refund you.*

thirty winning ways

1. Calorie balance
2. All calories are not equal
3. Need to move a bit
4. Grooving new habits
5. Get your head straight
6. Get a goal
7. Sleep better
8. Cut the sweet stuff
9. Crank up the veggies
10. Removing temptation
11. Managing hanger
12. Swapping the snacky habits
13. Sneaky exercise habit
14. Write it all down
15. Ride the endorphins
16. Make a commitment
17. Choose an inertia strategy
18. Intelligent food group choices
19. Get some help. Buddy up
20. Daily weights. Work a spread sheet
21. Enjoy food
22. Eat slowly
23. Nothing which needs a label
24. Would a caveman eat it?
25. Don't eat to fill an emotional hole
26. Set artificial rules
27. No bored snacking
28. No distracted eating
29. No procrastinating by eating
30. No sad snacks, no comfort binges
31. When you fall off the wagon

BetterNights

one
calorie balance

Calories in and calories out is a bit out of fashion at the moment. The truth is that although boring; it matters.

If you consistently eat less than you burn, you will lose weight. Period.

As with so many things in life, the whole picture is a bit more complicated. But *you* want results. *I* want you to get results. And that means having a daily negative calorie balance. This will mean some restriction of intake. It will mean some more burning by increasing your activity level. In short, upping your game a bit. Do this day after day and you will see the results.

They say that all good things come to those who wait.

What really happens is those who wait, gain weight. The reality is:

All good things come to those who work really hard at it.

Working hard at something brings its own rewards. It brings satisfaction. Our brains are hardwired to enjoy getting stuff done. This is handy.

We enjoy having stuff, but we enjoy it more if we've had a hand in its creation.

Flat-packed furniture, part-baked goods and cake mixtures are great examples of this. The companies know that psychologically we value something so much more if we've made it ourselves. When you add an egg, beat the mixture and put it in the oven for the correct time, you will enjoy what comes out much more than if you'd just bought it from a shop. You feel a sense of pride. A sense of ownership. The feel-good chemicals in your brain (mostly *dopamine* in this case) help you to feel self-satisfied and a bit smug.

The same applies to getting results in your life. Such as working on getting a better looking waistline. If you've had to work at these results a bit, you get to feel a whole lot better about yourself when you achieve them. So just because it can be a bit tricky to get a beach-ready body, don't be put off.

This is a good thing, because turning it around from where you are now is going to take a bit of effort and discipline. But it is **definitely do-able**. Start today, keep going tomorrow and then again the day after. You *will* start to see results, this brings its own rewards and the cycle continues.

Most of us have gained weight over the previous years. Bit by bit. It's not that we did anything very wrong on any one day. It is just that the accumulated excess has all added up too much. And the lottery of genetics is stacked against you.

Many of my patients tell me they do not over eat and that they eat less than their friends. This may be true. We all have a different *basal metabolic rate* - the amount of energy each of us burns is different. Some are lucky; they burn a lot, can eat a lot and don't become fat. The rest of us aren't quite so lucky.

This is of course a bit sad. But feeling sorry for yourself isn't going to change anything. The equation is simple. It is straightforward. If you eat a little more than you burn, you will put on weight. If you eat a little less you will lose it.

Many of my patients become disappointed, even despondent when their hard efforts don't seem to show results. They believe that somehow their body doesn't quite work *that* way and they put on weight due to unfortunate glands, or some such excuse. So here is a bit of a reality check. I **don't** want to be mean and **don't** want to put you off but I **do** want you to be realistic about what is likely to happen.

If you've gained weight over five years, why would you expect it to fall off in a few weeks? It will take a while. Most people can see a difference in a month. But not much before. And that is tough. I know. You work hard, but see nothing for many many days.

If you've gained an extra one hundred calories a day on average over ten years, that will be one hundred pounds. To lose this at the same rate will take ten years. But if you are in negative calorie balance every day of five hundred, you can lose about a pound a week. Losing more than this can be done, but not many of my patients keep this up for more than three months. I recommended aiming for just over a pound a week and keeping that going for as many months as you need. That means you are going to be wanting to be in negative balance of *more than five hundred calories nearly every day.*

Don't have too many off days.

Have a few days where you achieve more. You will soon enough see results even though they don't appear overnight. Watching the results and tracking what you do (*calories in, calories out, exercise done and daily weights*) each and every day will help to keep you on track and moving forwards. Even if you are on the right track, you need to be moving in the right direction and also moving fast enough so the coming train doesn't get you.

two
all calories are not equal

The way your body handles food is complex. Really complex. Confusingly, it also changes over time. It changes depending on your activity levels, it changes with the food habits you have and it changes depending on how much is in your fat stores.

It also changes with your muscle bulk, it changes with your age and it changes with your level of sleep. It changes when you are well and when you are sick. It definitely changes depending on what sort of foods you put in the top end. You burn calories simply by being alive. This is called your basal metabolic rate. It its a bit like your car engine when it is idling. Some cars idle faster than others. The brain needs to be powered, the liver needs to work, you need to generate heat, food needs digesting, you need to breathe and so on.

If you have a lot of protein and very few carbohydrates (carbs) in your diet, your body likes this. Your body can handle natural fats reasonably well as long as there aren't too many carbs. You can even lose weight while eating a high fat diet. But sticking to a high fat diet can prove tricky and getting it right is harder still. For a really simple set of rules to follow:

- Eat more protein.
- Eat more fiber (mostly from vegetables, from whole grains: have only have a very few, despite aggressive and misleading marketing).
- Cut all sugars. Yes all.
- Have fewer carbohydrates.
- Eat more veggies.
- If you hit a negative calorie balance each and every day, then natural fats are ok. If you cannot reliably do this, then cut the portion sizes of your fats right down to nearly zero.

Having enough protein will help keep your muscle bulk. Your muscles are vital for your weight loss plan. They will get you moving, make you feel better and will help prevent injuries.

The fiber will keep your bowels healthy. Your bowels are a series of long tubes of muscle. These contract to waft food from the top end towards the waste pipe. Fewer long term problem conditions develop, including cancer, if they have plenty of bulk to contract against. Carbohydrates and fat don't count as bulk as they are readily broken down to become soft and squishy. Protein counts, but fiber is better. Eat many grams a day. Vegetables are your best source of this.

Cut sugar from your diet. You don't need it. Eating food with sugar in it is not healthy eating. Sugary foods are laden with unhelpful calories and provide no useful nutrition. Cut as many as you can. Every day.

Have fewer carbohydrates. For the same reason as the sugars. Elite athletes need some carbs for intense cardio sessions to increase their VO_2 max. The rest of us don't really need them. At all.

Sure, they taste nice. Sure, we are used to them in the diet. But do you want to be thinner or not? Well, the more you cut, the better your chance of success. Your choice. But note that as many as two thirds of the population don't handle carbs well. The more carbs they eat, the fatter they become (belly fat, the worst kind). If you are reading this though, the odds are that you are one of these and should seriously consider cutting them down. A lot. It's up to you.

Eat more vegetables. A lot more. Most of my patients need to **quadruple** their intake. **4x**. I've said it before and will say it again. You'll eventually get bored of my nagging. But this is the quickest, cheapest, easiest way to become more healthy. Eat more and more and more.

As for the fats, until you get the hang of eating really, and I mean *really*, well - it is probably best to cut them right back. They contain massive numbers of calories and it is so easy to get this bit wrong. It's so easy to undo the good efforts and all the hard work you have put in elsewhere.

But they do taste nice. Perhaps limit yourself to a teaspoon of olive oil on your lunchtime salad.

three
need to move a bit

Whatever your current exercise level: Crank it up.

Really do this. Turn it up two notches this week. Next week turn it up again, and so on. Many of my patients come to me when they are stuck. Often they have a lot of pain in their knees, ankles and back. They cannot get out to jog for miles. If you can, you have few excuses not to.

If you are hampered by pain, then you will have to restrict your intake to achieve a negative calorie balance each day. Your task will be simpler if you get creative and burn some extra calories.

Try these:

- Put the TV remote far away, walk to it.
- Park at the far end of the car park.
- Don't use a shopping cart, carry a basket. Pay, take to car. Go back in and get your second basket.
- Have the heating down lower. You burn more calories in the cold. Take off a layer.
- Accidentally on purpose forget things around the house and have to go back to the other room to get them. This is even better if you go up and down stairs.
- Gently (or enthusiastically) dance to music while around the house. Bop to tunes while you are in your car.
- Fidget while watching TV. Really. Move your arms, legs and feet around. In studies done in old folks homes, those that fidget live years longer and die at half the rate than those who don't.

Some people are able to get out on their bike, get to the gym, get on the treadmill or run around on a local trail. If this is you, then do it.

You will soon reap the rewards. You will improve in fitness each and every day.

You will tone up and feel better. Eating better will become easier. You will burn more calories and the feel good chemicals released on sweaty exercise will give you an addictive boost.

For the rest of us too busy, too tired and too much in pain or unwell to do this, we will need to find different strategies. Be creative. Anything you can do which moves your body helps. The more the better.

Think about how you can change your daily routine. Tweak it and tinker to include more movement. What can you do? Sit up straight, get up out of the chair more often. Walk around the flat, the office, the shop, warehouse or wherever you happen to be. Can you take more trips, park further away, offer to fetch things for friends, colleagues and others?

Perhaps even try deliberately doing bicep curls with heavy items, triceps dips (easily done on office chairs) and squats (best performed when no one is looking). Can you work on your posture and tummy muscles while in queues, or stood on the train? Could you walk more briskly and upright? Could you carry the shopping a little further?

Write your successes down. When you write it down, you do stuff better. Each and every day try to out-perform what you did yesterday. Let me know what really works for you and the parts you feel smug about. Perhaps post about when it goes well on your blog, the book of faces, grinder or tinder.

four
grooving new habits

Habits are the stuff we do without thinking:

1. Doughnut in hand,
2. Put in mouth,
3. Repeat until all doughnuts gone.

That was your old habit. A better habit:

1. See doughnut,
2. Smile,
3. Pat slimmer tummy and reach for celery stick,
4. Munch,
5. Go for short walk,
6. Feel smug.

It would be really handy to have new helpful automatic behaviour patterns rather than the old unhelpful ones. But just like all habits, they aren't instantly changed.

However, work at them consistently and bingo, just like magic, they *will* become automatic.

■ Can you think of some unhelpful ones you have?
■ Which better ones would you like to replace them with?
■ How can you make a start?

Most of us drift through life on autopilot. This is quite natural. Autopilot uses less brain power. Literally. It actually uses less energy to produce our automatic behaviors. This is why they evolved.

They evolved so the power hungry brain used less energy. In life or death survival situations across thousands of generations, the early humans with better automatic behaviors tended to survive better.

And here we are in the 21st century. Doing stuff without thinking is usually helpful. It frees up our conscious brain to do more interesting stuff, like daydream, fantasize, or plan our next shopping trip.

The trouble with automatic decisions is that sometimes we want to do things differently. Like lose weight. If the autopilot reaches for the plate of pastries and not the carrot sticks, then we have a problem.

The great news is that **all** automatic behaviors can be reprogrammed. It takes a bit of concentration and effort. But can be done.

If your old behaviour was having cookies with your morning coffee break, you might want to have *no cookies* as your change of choice. You will need to use some willpower and start to do something different. This is a *pattern interrupt*. Your old behaviour followed a simple course and you need to derail it. Bump it off the tracks. Maybe have your drink in a different room. Sit in a different chair. Have a two minute walk and a glass of water instead of the coffee. Visit the restroom, then back to work with no cookie.

Like an old pair of shoes, your old habits feel comfortable. When you try on a new one for size, just like new shoes, they feel odd. After a while of persisting with your new shoes (and new habits) they become familiar and eventually they feel normal.

This process takes about two to six weeks for most people.

Less than forty two days to groove the new neural pathways in your brain. Don't worry if you have an off day. Simply do the new behaviour the next day. Just try not to have too many off days. It's like training a toddler or a puppy. Consistency is the key.

five
get your head straight

You need your body, mind and spirit to be all working in harmony.

I agree, that does rather sounds like a whole lot of woo (and I hate woo. This is a **proper** book grounded in **real** medical science). What I mean is that if you are stressed, tired, ill, have relationship stresses, a job you hate or money worries, then you aren't going to get your game-face on with your waistline. Your eye won't be on the ball and you will not get great results.

Until you get the rest of life as sorted as you can, you aren't going to get much slimmer. I see this a lot with my patients. That's the bad news, the good news is that once you start to be pro-active and straighten out these minor life wrinkles, the weight stuff is much easier to concentrate on.

Lots of my patients put on weight and then become sad, depressed and unmotivated. Lots of my patients are sad, depressed and unmotivated, they comfort eat to try and help. They put on weight.

It's a case of chicken and egg. What came first, the chicken or the egg? The answer is that there isn't really an answer but the answer doesn't actually matter that much. You should eat both the chicken and the egg (*they are high in protein, low in fat and contain no carbohydrates - a winning combination for your future healthy nutrition*).

Being a bit miserable, bored, out-of-sorts, down-in-the-dumps, or being in-a-funk goes hand in hand with eating junk food. I don't really care which bit leads to which. The point is that it happens often and needs a solution.

The solution, as with so many things in life isn't always straightforward. If it were, then none of us would end up with the problem in the first place. Any subject which has more than one expert and more than one book (weight management certainly counts), usually has no one single solution.

However, just because there is no one single solution, that doesn't necessarily mean that there isn't a way out for you. It's just that you will have to tailor-make your own out of the many available. This book has a whole bunch of differing approaches and I hope you can pick and choose to find your favourite.

To get your brain working with you rather than against you is crucial if you are going to shed pounds from your waist. Five steps today:

> **First:** acknowledge that sometimes your brain isn't helpful.

> **Second:** accept that you may have to try a few approaches before hitting the right one.

> **Third:** pick a big goal and go for it.

> **Fourth:** think of what brings you down. Write a list. Go through the list and try to minimise these, swap them, or try not to let them bother you so much.

> **Fifth:** Write another list, things that fulfill you and bring you up. Do more of these. Enjoy them more.

Remember to work your body and brain well to get the most out of them. The brain needs entertaining, then rest. Your body needs exercise, good fuel, than rest. This will help your mental brain relax and do all the right stuff. Just like the body, it repairs. The body repairs damaged tissue and the brain repairs damaged thoughts. It does its own restorative psychoanalysis each and every night.

It does this magic stuff while your conscious brain is sleeping. This is part of what dreaming is, along with creative thinking, complex problem solving and the fixing of your memories. Give your brain a chance to do its vital work, don't sedate it. Allow it to worry. You are allowed to give it a few nudges in the right direction. And just like any training: Note where you are, have a goal and aim better each time you check in. Congratulate yourself for any progress and then go back to the top of the cycle.

six
get a goal

Ok, I'm still going with these sports analogies. Get a goal, set a target, find an end point to aim at and focus all your efforts on this.

What motivating goal will work for you? I don't know, yet. Many of my patients choose things like wanting to be alive to see their grandchildren, wanting to be a size fourteen for next year's wedding, wanting to not be the fattest in family photographs at Thanksgiving, wanting to look hot in their red thong bikini at their next office party (I mean, next beach holiday).

Your target doesn't matter to me, but it has got to matter to you. Specific targets work best. Targets you can hold up (like '*I want to weigh one hundred and twenty pounds*'), compare where you are (*I weigh two hundred pounds*) and then compare the two. You then know this week isn't going to be the week you arrive and some more work is required.

If you have a vague goal ('*I want to be healthy and my knees to look nicer*') and look in the mirror, you won't know as easily where you are in relation to your grand goal and this can feel less motivating.

Our brains work better when they have stuff to do. Specific but achievable stuff. It is all about being whelmed:

Too much stuff = overwhelm = stress.
Too little stuff to do = underwhelm = boredom.

When we are stressed or bored, most of us tend to overeat. And we tend to overeat junk. It is in our best interests to have just the right amount and just the right sort of stuff to do.

Our unconscious brain filters out most of the billions of pieces of sensory information that floods into our brain each and every day. It presents just the right amount of information for us to cope with. This filtering process is subconscious. It happens without our thinking too much about it. We notice just the edited highlights. We receive terabytes of data daily from our eyes, our sense of touch, our tastebuds, our ears and noses bombarding us day in and day out. We notice some of it, we think about some of it and we remember some of it. An awful lot gets discarded.

Have you ever thought about how our unconscious brain decides what to show us and what not to, while sifting through all of this? It is a complex process and happens at nearly the speed of light. We don't know for sure about all of it, but modern neuroscience has discovered lots about these hidden processes.

We all have a mental list of goals and plans for the day. Our subconscious brain will help us to achieve these. It will be on the lookout for stuff which will help and opportunities. It will also try to identify threats which run counter. Interestingly we can direct these unconscious processes a bit. If we do not, the body and brain will drift on autopilot, mostly doing ok, but won't make much progress in any particular life direction.

If you buy a new car, in the months to come you will notice all the cars on the road the same make as yours. They were there previously, but your focused brain let them go by unnoticed. You can prove this in the comfort of your own chair where you are reading right now: Look around and notice everything green you can see. Notice any details and close your eyes and picture the green stuff, trying to recall the tiny details. Next, look around for everything brown or black. You will find yourself noticing detail in all your surroundings which passed by unnoticed only seconds earlier.

What has this got to do with weight loss? Good question. It is about having your goal and focus. Have a super-clear goal you can aim for. The rest of your brain will then be searching, on a daily basis for stuff to help you out (using the fancy *reticular activating system* if you want to get all technical). It will start to spot opportunities, things that support your progress, along with pitfalls and traps to watch out for. It will also start to notice fellow travelers on the same quest.

Having a clear set of goals also engages a fancy psychological trick. We are hardwired out of the box to stick to our beliefs. We will nearly always act in a way that is consistent with who we believe we are. If you believe you are a fat loser, you will probably stay one because your unconscious brain will let you drift along like that. I know this also sounds like woo, but a century of hard psychology science backs this up.

If you believe you are on a mission to shed pounds and become a happy healthy sexy human being, then your conscious brain will look out for stuff to help you. It will help you make decisions on autopilot that help you.

Your unconscious brain doesn't mind too much what your goals are, but once you have them nice and clear, like a faithful servant and cool high-tech futuristic robot, it will steer your towards your goals.

So choose them well, choose them carefully. Write them down. Start to believe you are progressing towards them and your unconscious brain will help you make some serious daily progress towards them. You still have to eat less and move more, but it is nice to know that your brain will be working with you and supporting you, rather than being a spare part, an unhelpful companion or a thing in the way.

seven
sleep better

When I'm tired I get grouchy and want to go piraña on snacks. I prowl the cupboards and eat anything in sight. There is a good biological basis for why I do this and I suspect you are wired up the same.

If you are tired, you aren't going to do well with weight loss. If you are tired every morning you are going to find each day quite tricky. With all grand plans, they need sticking at to get any decent results. This beach-ready body mission is no exception. Stick with it; you will win. Don't stick with it; you will lose.

So sticking with it each day would be good. To make this even a vague possibility, you are going to need to employ cunning tactics. **Sleep** is your cunning tactic of the day. It is one of my favorites. I like sleep. Having more makes me happy. It makes me less grouchy and altogether a bit more pleasant to be around (not great on most days if I'm honest).

If you work at getting at least eight hours (I'm serious, really eight hours) shut-eye each night, you will find it much easier to lose weight. Ignore this at your peril. I mean every night. You cannot bank this and store it up. You cannot catch up at a weekend by having lie-ins. They are nice, but only really repair the damage from the last couple of days. Nap in the afternoon if you need to, the more the better.

If getting off to sleep is a challenge, stop all of your caffeine for a few weeks, start a worry diary and turn off anything electronic for four hours before you go to bed.

Make sure you've had enough exercise during the day and follow the schedule in the BetterNights section at the back of this book if you need more tips.

If you are an oversleeper getting more than ten hours a night and can't get up in the mornings, then don't try to sleep more. You may be ill - see a doctor. You may have depression that is worth treating - also see a doctor. Until you iron out that particular wrinkle, the weight isn't going to shift much. That is the place to start for you.

Don't be afraid to nap. Having a short doze can revitalize you. It can energize you and lift your mood. If your mood is higher, you stand a much better chance of making better foody decisions.

A good night's sleep is the hallmark of champions.

eight
cut the sweet stuff

This is a story in two parts.

Part one: *If you eat sugar, you will become fatter.*

Sugars give a quick energy hit which we are driven by our biology to enjoy. So far, so good. But this sugar is rapidly absorbed into the blood stream and blood sugar levels rise. Because this is poisonous to the body we have a natural firefighting mechanism to bring this down to safe levels.

This is done by insulin release from our pancreas. Blood sugar is lowered by the action of insulin driving the glucose molecules into cells. Particularly fat cells. This is where our body stores energy. It very efficiently turns that sugar into fat ready to use on another occasion, just in case we need to run away from a saber-toothed tiger.

Sugar in the top end. Converted quickly to fat. All down to insulin. Insulin is released in tiny (safe) quantities until our blood sugar goes up and then our bodies makes oodles of it and pump it into the blood stream (in diabetes the insulin either doesn't get made very well - *type one* or the cells don't really listen to it anymore - *type two*).

Short version is no sugar = no insulin = no driver to fill up the fat cells.

If you want a less bulging middle, then don't let your sugar levels rise too quickly. This is achieved by eating less sugar, fewer carbohydrates (potato, rice, pasta, bread, cereals, grains) and more protein, fat and fiber. Did I say eat more fat? - yes, this will not cause your sugar levels to rise. In the bigger picture, remember fat is really high in energy density (calories) and if you want fewer calories in, you may want to go pretty easy on eating this, but a small amount will do you no harm, and possibly much less harm than eating sugary stuff.

Part two: *If you have a sweet tooth, this can be changed.*

The second part of the sweet stuff story is about not wanting to eat sweet stuff. I'm talking about having a sweet tooth. Having a sweet tooth means being used to having sweet stuff going in and if you don't have sweet stuff, you miss it. Some people eat veggies and love them, most people prefer candy. But the thing is, you can train your body in one direction or another. Always drink diet sodas and you will probably never lose your sweet tooth. While this gives no calories, you will always be at risk of making poor choices. This is because you are still treating yourself to a sweet tasting drink and getting your sweet fix.

Why not make it easier for yourself? I'm a big fan of making life easier.

This needs some actions and changing your old habits:

Plan: *Cut the sodas. You are not a child, it is time to ditch them and be all grown up about this. You can ignore me and call me an interfering idiot. That's ok - I'm* **not** *here to be your friend. I want you to get results and this is what you need to achieve them the fastest. It works, so go with this one.*

Plus - fruit juices are sweet, so don't drink them. Period. Not ever more. Just stop. They are laden with sugar (even if it goes by the fancy name fructose) and I don't care if they make you feel healthy. Stop, right now.

nine
crank up the veggies

Q. What is the difference between vegetables and booger snot?
A. Small boys won't eat vegetables.

Handily, you aren't six years old anymore. So there is no longer any excuse. You are a grown up and it is now time to eat like one.

Getting a *beach-body* or a *I-look-good-in-a-mirror-naked* body that you are proud of, relies on doing everything so far. And doing it well. You then need to fuel your body well. To fuel this magnificent body of yours, to give you a healthy glowing skin and to simply ooze raw sex appeal you will need to select your foods carefully. If you had a Formula-One racing car or a thoroughbred stallion, you would not put junk in. You would not settle for anything other than the very best.

Having invested so much time, energy and practice exercise sessions you want it to fire on all-cylinders and be in tip-top condition. For this my friend we turn to salads and vegetables. Even fruit. That's pretty much it. Some meat, cheese, chicken, fish, eggs, nuts, legumes and pulses will help - but it's mainly about fresh veggie stuff. As much as you can manage. Your vitamin levels will soar. Your fiber content will be perfect. Your bowels will be magnificent (that's a good thing) and your body will be healthier and trimmer than ever before. What more could you possibly want for as you contemplate your magnificence in the full length mirror of your choice.

Imagine you've just met the lover of your dreams and they've turned up at your place breathless and willing. Dressed to thrill, stood in front of you getting hot, steamy and ready. You've just polished off a bread and butter pudding with custard, followed by cheesecake, a couple of doughnuts and an ice cream milkshake with whipped cream. Even the goddam cherry on the top. Plus the hundreds and thousands. And the chopped nuts. Even the warm buttery toffee sauce. After a full dinner with starters, soup, roll, salad and main course. That encounter is not going to be quite as good as you were hoping for.

Fuel your body well. Vegetables and stuff with vitamins. Plenty of fiber too. Hopefully you'll also avoid the overeating scenario above.

Having two pieces of fruit a day is about the right number. Fewer than this and you may become deficient in vitamins. Particularly vitamin C. This will help you not to get *scurvy*. You really don't want scurvy if you are going to impress people. Your hair falls out and grows back all funny, your gums swell and your teeth fall out. You have low energy and on the whole don't look too impressive.

So, listen up and eat fresh fruit. This will also give your bowels a workout. A workout for my bowels I hear you cry? - quite right. That fiber stuff is pretty important. It doesn't count if you have fruit juice. Juicing is a stupid idea. It is fashionable right now. But that doesn't make it a good idea (*a bit like colonic irrigation*). Juicing removes all of the lovely fiber from a nutritious set of ingredients. You aren't a child, man up and eat the whole fruit or veg. It's much better for you. Your gut walls get to clench down on some substance. This is thought to help prevent bowel cancer and that can only be a good thing. It also will help you have nice predictable well formed solid poops. And who doesn't feel better after a good poop? This is all about feeling better, looking better, feeling fitter and I reckon you can make a good start from the inside out.

Back to the fruit. If you have more than the two pieces I've just recommended you hit the curve of diminishing returns. Too much fruit and you will poop too much. It will become all runny and there is no telling when an inconvenient follow-through moment might materialize. Plus, if you have lots of fruit, it is not without its calories. Each piece of fruit contains just about 100 calories. This is ok if you are in good shape, stick to two a day and are getting a decent workout each day. If you are gulping down four or five pieces each day, you are going to possibly be overdoing it on the calorie front and are certainly getting too many carbs to aid your developing beach-ready body. If you want your abs to show up and impress people, you are going to need to dial back on the carbs. I don't care what you've read about fruit being of the unlimited variety of good food, this is where we are at. Two pieces a day. That's it. Got it? Good.

Did I mention veg? You can't get enough veg. Eat plenty, they have vitamins, they taste yummy, you will lose flab and will become healthier. Really, eat more. Quadruple your intake. It's really good for you.

ten
removing temptation

"I can resist everything apart from temptation."

Oscar Wilde, Lady Windermere's Fan, 1892, Act I

Quite: Me too.

But to make decent progress you are going to have to eat better stuff. You are going to need to make great choices. All day. Every day. And then do it all over again the next day.

Temptation is the desire to do something. Particularly something unwise or forbidden.

There are **two parts of our brain** that are in constant battle. The *animal brain* which we share with the animal kingdom and the *human brain* which we evolved after our separation from the other animals.

The **animal brain** keeps us safe, fights other animals and tries to find, impress and reproduce with the best possible mates. Then it tries to protect our offspring as this is in our own genetic interests. This is the part of the brain which gives us strong emotional drives if it thinks there are any of these tasks to be done. It thinks in the here and now and doesn't think too much about the consequences. This is the part of the brain which seeks cake and chocolate. This brings comfort and plentiful calories: Which it thinks are important for survival.

The newer **human part of our brain** is the so-called clever part. This does complex thinking about planning an organizing. This is the one which gets you ready for work in the morning. This one saves for a retirement fund. This is the one that keeps you socially aware at a dinner party. This helps us fit into society and enjoy the economic and social benefits such as hospitals, fire brigade, and police who try to keep us all safe.

The human brain is the one who will work to get you fit again and will be doing the hard work of keeping you to task if you are on a mission for a beach-ready body.

The human brain will have to contend with fighting the urges and the desires of the animal brain. The animal brain will always be there. The voice of temptation which usually wins if you aren't concentrating or are tired. We will have to play to the strengths of the human brain if we are going to make any progress. I suggest treating the animal brain like an unruly toddler. You can give it love, but to stop it ruling the house you will have to set and stick to some rules. You will have to use cunning and sometimes distract it. You will need to think of tricks that stop the animal brain doing its thing and driving you to constantly graze, just in case there is a famine coming.

The human brain is smarter and knows there is no famine. But cunning tactics are needed.

Well, they aren't that complex, but you need to be vigilant. With yourself.

Put temptations out of sight.

Hide the chocolate. Have no snacks in the house. Don't carry cash or cards so you can't just swing by the convenience store to pick up more snacks. Do hard exercise - the animal brain will be fooled into thinking you are running towards something important and it will drop your pain levels, increase your pleasure and stop yammering in your ear about finding snacks to eat. It will relax and enjoy the exercise with you. And it will even go quiet for ages afterwards, which can be super-helpful if you are trying to shovel less calories in the top end on any given day.

Outsmart the animal brain:
- *hide the snacks*
- *make it difficult to source more snacks*
- *keep really busy*
- *do hard exercise*

eleven
managing hanger

Hanger. This is being angry when you are hungry.

Usually this is something you notice in other people.

When people are running low on physical or mental reserves, they are grumpy and will verbally lash out at you, reject your advances and are generally not much fun to be around. Some days that might describe you. When you are hungry, you aren't yourself. Well you are, but not usually the side you want on public display.

To avoid hanger:

- **You can** time your food better by eating little and often.
- **You can** alter the content of your food. More fiber, more protein, fewer carbohydrates (which you burn through way too quickly. Think coals on the barbecue not just lighter fluid).
- **You can** plan not to be around others when you are at risk of hanger.
- **You can** consider small, low calorie healthy snacks to tide you over until your next meal.

Some people extend the hanger definition to include the states when people are most at risk of snacking. People trying to do without drugs or alcohol when they are battling addiction are told about *HALT*.

HALT is what they are supposed to do when they feel vulnerable and alone and want to reach for the drugs. They are supposed to *stop and think* about what they are about to do. They then find another solution with doesn't involve the drugs. The same thing applies to snacking. When you are feeling hangry; stop and think. Don't go and snack. **HALT** stands for **H**ungry, **A**ngry, **A**lone, **T**ired. If this applies to you; Stop. Think about what you can do to feel better which doesn't involve a family sized bucket of anything, then go and do it. Minimize the calorie load during your temporary crisis.

You can choose to get around hanger by prevention or cure. Prevention is always better than a cure.

If you ignore hanger, you run the risk of being crabby, crotchety and unpleasant to be around if you get hungry. If you are serious about doing something about your expanding waistline, you are probably going to feel hungry on occasion. Hunger isn't bad for you, but it is a powerful sensation. This is the animal part of your brain telling you to go and find food. To kill for it and trample anyone in your way if necessary. It is no wonder that a few tempers fray when part of us thinks it is starving.

But hunger is like an over-sensitive car alarm or a smoke detector that goes off whenever you make toast. You know there is no emergency and you have the situation under control, but there it is beeping and chirruping away to tell you *'the end of the world is nigh'* and to *'panic, panic, panic'*.

Ideally you will want to turn down the sensitivity on the alarm. It has good intentions and is only trying to keep you safe. It doesn't know that there are nearby shops laden with calories and that your belly has enough stores to keep you going for weeks. All it knows is that you've not put any food in the top end for a few hours and it had got pretty used to you grazing all day, every day. So it thinks: *'what is going on? I must be starving. Panic, panic, panic. Go and kill for food. It is them or us!'*

To prevent hanger you need to eat little and often. To cure hanger, you need to be alert to it and respond in a calm and sensitive way. Be calm and measured while your inner animal is running around in a blind panic. Don't take it out on whoever is in front of you. There is no point yelling at traffic. There is little benefit in hitting the computer when it doesn't do what you want.

Got hanger? Calm down. Maybe eat a little something. Stop (HALT). Are you actually a bit hungry, angry, alone and tired? If so, what can you do right now which will remedy one or more of those feelings? Preferably choose one without calories. An ideal one is hitting the mental snooze alarm by going for a five minute walk or get on with a different task.

twelve
swapping the snacky habits

Find something to do with your hands. Reading, writing, typing, crocheting, knitting, needlepoint, playing an instrument. Preferably not chain smoking - but you need to be busy.

I prefer running at a decent pace - too fast to eat. Any exercise that leaves you out of puff makes it too hard to eat. If you can only manage a walk, then the key is not to take any snacks with you. You won't die of becoming hypoglycemic if you are out for less than twelve hours. Sure, you'll be a bit peckish and your tummy will grumble at you, but you will come to no harm.

We habitually snack. If this isn't you, then great. Skip to the next chapter. But for the rest of us, we've got into the behaviour pattern of cows and horses. Anything that grazes wanders around with its head to the ground chomping on anything tasty it can find. All the time when it has nothing better to be doing (running around, making babies and so on).

When we have nothing more pressing to be doing, we usually reach for whatever food is at hand. If there are chips, peanuts, pistachios, cookies, pretzels, gummy bears, jelly babies or doughnuts within arms reach we reach for them. Every time we wander past the snack bowl we will grab some. We usually don't even notice we are doing it. If we do, we justify it to ourselves saying that the handful only contains a few calories, so what harm can it do?

What harm can it do? If you eat only one hundred calories a day extra (a handful of snack) for ten years, you will gain one hundred pounds of fat (7.5 stones, 47 kilos). I reckon that is too much for just one handful. Just one handful. Assuming that for the other hours of the 3650 days of those ten years you were in perfect calorie balance, with no off-days.

Snacking then is a risky thing. But how can we change it? We all do it. And we are eating ourselves slowly to death.

The trick is in having a mental alarm bell. When you spot yourself doing it, stop. Just that once. These single episodes of stopping start to add up. Reach for the snack, stop the pattern, smile, pat yourself on the back for noticing. Be strong. Resist just this once. Get to feel smug.

Do this again and again. Maybe even tell someone you resisted. To groove a new habit takes most people between fourteen and about sixty days. During this time it feels different. That is ok, it is just your brain learning new stuff. But you have to persist.

If you can find yourself things to busy yourself with, this will help. Distract yourself. Chew sugar-free gum, rinse with disgusting mouthwash frequently. Do ten squats. Do something different. Swap those snacky habits.

thirteen
sneaky exercise habit

Exercise is good. Exercise makes you fitter, stronger, happier and healthier. It tones and firms your muscles, it burns calories, it gives you an addictive endorphin rush.

Yet many of us don't do it. We avoid it. We think it might hurt, make us sweat, look out of breath and we don't want people to stare at us when we wobble past.

But help is at hand. I invented *sneaky exercise* for just this very situation. Ok, I might not have invented it, but the name is mine. The concept is this: **The more exercise you do the better**. Any movement will help. They all use muscles and all burn calories. Cram as much as you can into the life you have already.

Sneak it in before your unconscious brain has a chance to raise any objections. **Sneak stuff in every day**. Tweak your normal day to day activities and generate new, helpful habits:

- Park at the far end of the grocery store car park.
- Always walk the stairs, never get in an elevator.
- Keep the TV remote on the TV, not the sofa.
- Get up to change the channel or the volume.
- Drink extra fluid and keep running up and down to the bathroom.
- Shopping baskets not carts. Use ten trips if you need to.
- If you forget something and need to go back for it, even back up stairs, don't curse; smile. That is a sneaky extra few calories. Your muscles will be better for it. You don't even need to tell anyone.

The benefits of **sneaky exercise** are in the calories burned. Not many, but they all count and soon add up. Burn enough calories and you will lose weight if you control what goes in the top end. Every calorie you burn counts. Calories burned in exercise have the bonus benefit of working your muscles. The better shape your muscles are in, the better your posture, wellbeing and resistance to infections and even cancer.

The key to **sneaky exercise** lies in the ability to do more and more each day, without much mental resistance. No one can object to walking a few extra paces each day. So if it is easy to do, you might be more likely to try it. When my patients try it, they find it works. It isn't too much bother and can be done every day. Each and every day. Again and again.

Just the same as we damage ourselves by eating a few extra calories each day, we can slowly reverse this by doing the opposite. This is where **sneaky exercise** comes in. This is your human brain using its cunning to sneak exercise past the animal brain which might be selling you the misleading message of wanting to laze around and conserve calories *just in case* there is a famine coming. There isn't. If there really is, you should probably put this book down and do more important stuff in preparation for the impending apocalypse. Still here? Good. No famine coming then. So get off your butt and do some *sneaky exercise*.

The endorphin benefits of exercise also give you a little buzz when you complete any task. Even sneaky exercise. Strictly speaking, biochemically it's more like a dopamine rush (they are more addictive and that can only be a good thing). The fact is doing stuff feels good. Do it. Do more of it. Start today. Feel smug. Write it down. Feel more smug. Same again tomorrow. Well done you.

fourteen
write it all down

Writing stuff down keeps you on task. The act of being observed alters the observed act. This is widely misquoted and mis-attributed as being the *Heisenberg uncertainty principle* (the observer effect is correcter). Heisenberg was a clever physicist who made some astounding predictions about subatomic particles in 1927 which paved the way in quantum mechanics and are applicable to all wave-like systems. Most people simply know him as a fictional wayward chemistry teacher.

Your beach-ready body mission will be aided well by utilizing the less famous *Hawthorne effect*. In Hawthorne in 1924, the Western Electric Works did some experiments to find out how to increase widget production. They measured widgets made and varied the conditions; more light, less light, messy work place, tidy work place. They found that widget production went up with more light, but also less light and it even improved if they simply had no change in the condition.

Work rate went up for all conditions. They concluded that being measured and observed makes you work a bit harder. Not really rocket science (like that Heisenberg chap) but it was revolutionary in its day.

Measure something, you do it better. It's all about concentration and focus. Again, not really much of a brain science mystery but underestimated in its power.

It's really powerful. Write stuff down. Write what you eat. Write what you do. It is right to write it all down. Every day.

The Hawthorne effect in action is seen when we write down what we do. Well researched, it applies to so many things in life. This is one of them. It applies to and is effective for exercise and for food intake. I also use it for my biggest patients when tailor-making their weight programs. Elite athletes use it for their weight too - I'm a fan of that.

Daily stuff, check in each morning - this is when hope and motivation are at their highest. Each morning, you get a brand new dose. Our brains like to be busy. Not too busy, that is overwhelm. But just enough busy to stop us daydreaming. We like to break the day up into small manageable chunks and do one thing at a time. When we do this, we feel more contented. If we feel more contented, we tend to snack less.

Having our human brain in charge will help stop the animal brain from taking over and driving us to seek food and lie about. Part of being in charge of your day using the conscious brain means giving it something to aim at. This is why goals are good. Keeping it on task is the next challenge.

Daily check ins and reassessment of how you are doing compared to your goals is *really* useful. Having a self-assessment question helps:

What did I do today to move me towards one of my goals?

The idea here is that you get to answer with something positive each day. And if you can't, that gives you a mental kick up the rear to make sure that as you drift off to sleep you are planning cunning strategies to rectify this the next day.

This simple act of writing will help you make progress more than anything else. Plus, it's easy. But you do have to actually do it (not just nod and smile). Don't be fooled by the apparent simplicity of it. I'm right. Write. Get a pen. Do it. Every day.

fifteen
ride the endorphins

When you do stuff you feel good. When you make a cake you feel good (eating is nice too but it tastes nicer if you've made it). Self assembly furniture, part baked goods: They all use the psychological mind tricks of achievement.

You can use this too. You need to work out where the buzz is and what you need to do to trigger it. Then do more of it. Do stuff each day that uses these cunning tricks to fool your animal brain.

Your body and brain (the unconscious part) makes lots of chemicals in the background and releases these at what it thinks is just the right time. These then give you powerful feelings. When you are tiring while doing important exercise (running away from an angry mammoth), adrenaline is released giving you a powerful burst of energy, drive and renewed enthusiasm for running away. Tiredness is banished and you are able to think more clearly as well as run away at your top speed.

Similarly, if you are chasing down prey across the grasslands and some of your joints or muscles hurt, endogenous morphine-like substances (*endorphins*) are released and you forget about or can ignore the pain. This enables you to catch the prey so you and your tribe can survive the coming winter.

Exercise releases endorphins (helps decrease pain and gives a high) and also a dopamine surge (feel-good chemical buzz and also a happy high). This is the stuff swishing around your brain when you are deep in infatuation.

Finishing tasks also releases dopamine, making us feel self-satisfied. A warm, fuzzy internal mental glow. This makes you want to do more of that sort of thing. All these chemicals are inbuilt. We can tap into them deliberately even though we aren't usually hunting or being hunted with our lives at stake.

Having a **to-do** list can weigh heavy on your mind. But having a **done** list is liberating. So replace your growing to-do list with a **done** one.

The trick to a done list is to put a lot of (easy) stuff on it.

<u>Less good</u>:
   1. *I'd like a pay rise next year* - you might not get it and you might have a long time to wait. The secret here is to set the bar **really low**.

<u>Why not try</u>:
   1. *Getting out of bed before the third snooze alarm* - tick.
   2. *Getting dressed* - tick.
   3. *Managing a light breakfast* - tick.
   4. *Smiling at one person* - tick.
   5. *Walking an extra five steps in the morning* - tick.
   6. *Sitting up straight at least once in the day* - tick.

…And so on. Write them all down. They all count (a little). These small victories add up. You will feel better. This will motivate you to do more stuff. As you make progress, shift your own goal-posts for what gets you a tick in the box. You are in charge. You are in control. Work it so that you make progress and get to feel good about it. Every day. This is the way forward. Stop beating yourself up with a to-do list. Have a done-list. Use those happy chemicals.

There are also feel-good chemicals which help us when we are hungry. If we are hungry, the body thinks we are starving to death and is motivated to go and find food rather than being programmed to lie down and accept it. So it doesn't always feel bad to be a bit hungry and your body and brain function perfectly well when you are. Many people feel mistakenly that they can't cope with what they feel is hypoglycaemia - this is of course rubbish in day to day situations. If you've just run a marathon and not eaten anything, then maybe you could have mildly low blood sugar. If you are on medicines which drop your sugar, then yes. Otherwise, no. Not so. That is a trick of the imagination. Learn what it feels like and you can then safely ignore the unhelpful hunger signals and get on with your day.

Did you know that hunger rises to a certain point, then doesn't escalate?

I always used to think that it just kept increasing until, until… I don't really know what I was expecting to happen. You don't explode, turn green or collapse dramatically. All that happens is you eat something - a normal amount and then you feel full and carry on as normal. It is almost disappointing. A bit of an anti-climax, but nothing much happens. So the upshot of this is that you really can skip meals or eat very little and no harm will befall you.

There are of course the caveats here that if you are pregnant, breastfeeding, have a (very very) rare metabolic medical condition or are on diabetic medications that lower your blood sugar - such as *gliclazide* or *insulin*, be careful. If that is the case - then don't do the *starving-yourself-a-bit* thing. Consult your doctor if you aren't sure. But most people can suck up a bit of hunger with no ill effects. You lose weight faster and it is good to learn where the full point is.

Most people's calibration is a bit wrong and we think we are much hungrier than we really are. It is well worth trying to find out where your actual set-point is.

Your plan: learn to be a bit hungry on occasion and do things, lots of them. Simple daily stuff. Do it. Give yourself a pat in the back. Feel good. Do it again. This will boost your happy thoughts and give lots of motivating releases of those happy chemicals (dopamine surges) in your brain

You then feel better able to handle what the day throws at you and can better deal with what the universe has in store without reaching for the comfort snacks.

sixteen
make a commitment

To commit is a to make a pledge. A pact. A promise. This can be something you make to yourself. We are hardwired to be true to our beliefs. We follow our own moral code. We defend our position, however sensible it is. We even defend ourselves if whatever we decide has become out of date, outmoded, or simply ridiculous.

It is all about saving face. This face saving is to do with survival in groups. We needs an amazing public persona to be strong. This is important to signal to others our status. It doesn't really matter if you *actually* have status or power. The important thing is to show it off to others. And this means saving face. You have to not only be a person of principles (ideals you believe in and stick up for) but you also have to demonstrate this to your group. This is fundamental psychology, we all do it.

We basically always try to show off a bit to impress rivals for food, resources and potential mates.

We care what others think about us.

The knock on of all this psychological talk is that when we make a commitment to ourselves, we stick to it pretty well. If we make this declaration out loud and in public, we are even more compelled and motivated to follow it through. Handily we can use this and harness it. We can learn to channel it for our own nefarious purposes.

I see this with my patients who attend diet groups - public declarations of weight losing abound. Also when people commit to do a sponsored race or event.

The good news is that your animal brain will blindly follow whichever pattern is programmed and your human conscious brain can choose these patterns at will. So if you decide to be an athlete, move like an athlete, get the waistline of an athlete and tell people you are on this mission; your unconscious decisions and public actions will start you on this path. Other people then start to help you. They will help by encouragement, trying to spot your progress and will gently tease you if you aren't quite up to speed. You never know, you may even inspire a few of them to follow in your footsteps and join you on the journey.

This is about consistency, self image and saving face. Decide you are going to do this. Manage your weight. Have better waist management. Cut the flab, tone up. Go for buff, become trimmer.

Whatever it is for you. Just decide. Decide comes from the Latin *de-* from and *cadere* meaning to cut off. Literally cut off your other options. Once you've decided. Be true to yourself. Tell other people and ask them to keep you on track. Make yourself accountable to them. Get a weight loss buddy.

Tell everyone, post on *Facebook*. Get a *Strava* account. Publish your weights and how you are achieving them. Tell other people what is working and the days you find hard. When it goes wrong, 'fess up. Correct the wobble and get back on track. Everyone loves a winner. But more people love the underdog story. If you've tried, failed, tried, failed, picked yourself up, given yourself a good talking to and come through the other side of your dark place: Now, *that* is a story to tell. That is what makes a Hollywood blockbuster and will impress anyone you want. True grit.

If it were easy, it would impress no one and more people would look like models. But most of us are too round. So, decide today. Write it down. Shout it out loud and proud. Commit to the new you. Start today. Get on with it. What are you waiting for? You owe it to your future self.

Decide. Cut off all other options from your future. Decide and commit.

Decide = from French décider, from Latin decidere *(to determine)*, from de = off + caedere = cut.

Today's action: *make your public promise. Make it big and bold. Put out the banners. Tell everyone you meet and put a deadline on the calendar. Put up posters in your workplace and get people to track your progress with you.*

seventeen
choose an inertia strategy

Overcoming inertia proves tricky for many people. Getting going. How to do it? Things in motion tend to stay in motion, but things at rest, tend to stay at rest. This physical law of the universe seems to apply to couch potatoes too. There seem to be two main helpful options which work really well. Your choice. Out of two: *Go big or go small.* Get into action though. Your choice is in quite how to get started. The phrase *'**just do it**'* is a great one (JFDI). It tells you how it is. If you want or need to get into action there is but one choice:

Do it. Or do not.

Choose to *do it* every time. Putting it off is a natural tendency - mainly because we are afraid of committing ourselves to a course of action we can't follow through. This fear is natural. Our emotions very much want us to have this public consistency and to be able to save face when we can. But this is a myth, a social construct. It is basically a rule we made up and isn't useful all the time.

Override this face saving rule. Get into action. I agree with what you are probably saying in your head: *it isn't always that easy doc.* True, it isn't always that easy. No it isn't and I agree with you.

But the way forward is **not** to sit and think about *what if, what if, what if.* Thinking of all the things that *might* happen if you *do* stuff. If you are going to do that you should add in the what-ifs of if you *don't* do stuff. These include; early death, daily pain from arthritis, early heart attacks and strokes from diabetes and much more importantly, a decrease in your sex-life enjoyment.

So if you are going to do something, just how do you go about that? How do we overcome this sitting around and whining about it that so many of us do? That is a good question and the best answer is:

Go large or go home.

This is a way of overcoming inertia. Inertia is a physical law of the universe (Newton's first law if you want to get technical). It states that if something is still, it stays still until you move it. And if it is moving it keeps going until something stops it.

If you have a weight-loss plan and it is going well it is much easier to keep this going than it is to get started in the first place. You may already have noticed this. This makes sense, so isn't exactly rocket science (though Isaac Newton's laws of motions from 1687 are the science that puts rockets into space. So actually it is rocket science).

Overcoming inertia (the tendency to sit on your ass eating cookies) can be done in two ways that work well:

Big or small. You get to choose.

The great big, kick up the ass method is probably the best. This fits in with the public commitment and means taking massive steps into action. Start big and carry on. Make a big commitment and then the only way you can actually achieve this is that everything else in your life has to take second place. Those things are then in the background of your major mission.

Understandably a few people quail at the thought of that (which is the whole point). That's ok, but a bit wussy. For those folk, the tiny baby-step approach might be a better fit. This softly softly approach is a daily extra tiny thing that gets snuck in without being big enough to object to. The trick is to add to it each and every day.

Softly softly take ten extra steps today. Tomorrow add in another ten. You can't object to that. Who could? Before too long you are hiking extra miles around town, just to get your step count up for the day. Leave an extra forkful on your plate. Take one spoon less desert. Before long your meals look more like they belong to someone with a developing beach-ready body than the plate of something that Greenpeace might harpoon on a beach.

We call this progress.

eighteen
intelligent food group choices

Eat well. Choose your food intelligently. We are all told this. But just what exactly does that mean? The books, magazines, newspapers and the internet tell us something new every day. The mountains of information, much of it contradictory sometimes seem insurmountable. We end up ignoring it. Even the good advice.

Here is today's plan, this week's strategy: Cut the carbs. Crank up the protein. Eat natural fats only. Use them for flavor, count them carefully and eat nothing fried.

All the food we eat gets broken down and processed. The plate might seem stuffed full of complex flavors, tastes, textures and colors. But once it gets past your throat on its way to becoming poop at the other end, your body doesn't care about any of that.

Your body only really cares about the major food groups, vitamins and minerals.

The major food groups are protein, fat and carbohydrate. Along with indigestible fiber and water these make up 99.99% of what you put in the top end. Vitamins are a handful of molecules your body can't make for itself from breaking down protein, fat and carbohydrate. The main ones are vitamins A, B, C, D, E and K.

Minerals are important but only really iron matters. The others are important but your body is so good at extracting these when it finds them, you can safely ignore them for probably your entire life on this planet. Iron is needed for healthy red blood cells. These transport oxygen. Iron is bountiful in green leafy vegetables and red meats. It is best absorbed with vitamin C (also in green leafy vegetables - unless you boil them in water. It leaks out into the water, which most of us pour away).

Back to our major food groups. Protein contains the building blocks of life. If you have enough you will be healthy. If you don't have enough your muscles will fade, you will feel tired and become less healthy.

It is a complete no-brainer to have lots of **protein** in your diet. Most of us don't get enough protein when we try to diet for weight loss. We follow some misleading information and try to eat heart-healthy carbohydrates. This is based on twenty years of public programs which have perhaps been a bit misdirected. Take it from me - **have enough protein**. You will see visible progress and will feel better. Then you will trust this program.

Fats? Fats is a complex one. Well not very complex, but easy to get a bit wrong. Fats have oodles of calories and give lots of energy. This is great if you are hiking solo across the Antarctic, but less helpful if you are trying to shed flabby pounds before your next sunnier holiday.

It used to be thought, twenty or so years ago, that eating fat caused higher cholesterol levels and gave you heart disease. We now know it is a lot more complicated than this and eating fats doesn't really do that. Being fat makes heart disease worse but eating it doesn't seem to make very much difference at all. If you have lots of fat in your diet you will clearly be having lots of high energy dense food. If you aren't burning it, your body will store it. In your fat cells. Most of us have too much energy in these stores and need to burn through it, rather than eating more of it.

Some fats are essential for life and people panic about getting the right amount. Actually you hardly need any of these and your body is great at extracting the ones you need. As long as you don't try to go completely fat-free you will be fine. I recommend having some fats in your diet but not thinking too much about them. Don't add them. But don't get obsessive if a few sneak in. Then that will be about right.

A lot is said about heart-healthy fats and omega numbers. A lot of people are making a lot of money rabbiting on about the benefits of some fats over others and selling expensive supplements. If these worked they would be free with healthcare. They aren't. The short version is that most of the science doesn't make much difference in real life. Only in test tubes. You can probably ignore most of the advertising advice and never need supplements

All fats are high in calories. Low fats spreads are also high in calories - compare them to olive oil and butter. Olive oil is probably all you need. If you have oily fish in your diet along with olive oil you will do really well and get just the right amount. If in doubt - don't have anything man made. And never fry anything. Frying stuff burns the fats and this makes them much worse for you.

Although probably the fat best for you, olive oil still has 40 calories in a single teaspoon (and 234 in a Mars bar).

I've left **carbohydrates** for last as there is a lot of bad information out there in the world. Carbohydrates include sugar, cereals, wheat, bread, rice, pasta, potatoes and root vegetables. These are plant stores of energy. As humans we do not need these. These have only been in our diet in quantity for the last twelve thousand years. This is about four hundred generations. That is all. We've been around as a separate species for 200,000 years. That is a long time for us to evolve without any carbohydrates in significant quantities. We do very well without them. But they are cheap and easy to make and grow in the 21st century.

Because of this, we eat a lot of them. The problem is that if we stuff our diets with these energy rich carbohydrates we don't eat enough protein. We sometimes miss out on vitamins. We then have too much energy around which our body stores as fat. In case there is a famine. But there is no famine, so we stay fat. Then we die young and so on.

If you cut back your carbohydrates you will feel better, you will eat into your fat stores more easily and will make much more progress than if you change any other part of your diet. Start today - cut out all sugars. That is the best place to start.

nineteen
get some help. Buddy up

- Going it alone can work.
- But having a pal, friend, buddy, chum, or partner in crime works just soooo much better.
- You can encourage each other.
- You will be accountable to each other.
- You will support and encourage the other one. They will do the same for you.
- You will share your journey with them, you can try and compete against them.
- You can whinge at them when it is hard and you can tell them to get a grip and refocus when they slide a little.
- You can tell them what is working for you and where your weak spots lie.
- Go shopping with them and help them make better choices.
- Go to the gym together, go swimming.
- Go jogging, long walks, borrow a dog if you need to.
- Go cycling, go to *Zumba*, yoga or salsa together.
- Be a team. A team of two.
- Double trouble and twice as fun.

Sometimes staying on track can prove tricky. Having a public commitment helps to a degree. Being motivated helps. Having a great target helps. Writing stuff down, keeping track and counting your progress all help. Having someone to keep close scrutiny on you helps even more. This can be someone you know or a stranger. It can be someone you see in person or someone online. They can live in your house, be someone you occasionally meet or they can live on the other side of the world.

Sharing this journey is a massive help. Find someone. Someone to encourage and cajole you. Someone who is also going through the same thing. A shared journey will throw up all sorts of help for the challenges and speed bumps you encounter from time to time. They can help keep you on target and moving in the right direction. Ask for help and advice. People love to give help and advice.

And in return you can provide help and advice. You can help them out. This feels good. This is a cunning way of reinforcing the identity of yourself as a person on journey towards a better beach-ready body with a booty to be truly proud of.

Teaching someone else what works for you is a great way of teaching yourself. You will find out what you *really* know and what you need to know more about. Sorting the hard facts from the woo or the advertising *bs*. You will find by teaching someone, by giving them tips that your understanding deepens. This is good thing.

If you have no friends or supportive partner, try chat rooms, special interest groups and look on the book of faces. As always, stay safe online. If you aren't sure of what that is, *Google* it. You need to know this stuff.

twenty
daily weights

Work a spreadsheet. Fill it out. Every day.

Some of my patients have a psychological blind spot with weight. I'm talking about the actual number. Pounds, stones, kilos, whatever. They have a bit of a freak out when they see how much they weigh. It is just a number, but I know some people have lots of associations and emotions that they have tied or anchored to this number. If that is you that is fine, but you should probably skip to the next chapter.

Still here? Good.

Daily weights. A Good thing. For most people. This is why:

Our brains are geared to make comparisons. We notice contrasts in all of our senses and the thought patterns on the inside mirror these. Meaning, you notice when there is a difference. And when there is not. Get a daily check-in and you will have a better daily bench mark.

Your weight will fluctuate on a day-by-day basis up and down. If you are gaining weight or if you are losing weight, this will happen over weeks, months and longer. The daily fluctuations are on top of this long term trend. You are interested in the long term trend. If you have only a few data points (weekly or monthly weigh-ins), you run the risk of these not giving you accurate numbers to contrast your feedback.

Your weight will go up a little bit with each meal and each drink, it will go down a bit with each visit to the bathroom and if you've not had a drink recently. It will change depending how much poop you have in your bowel at any one time and this can vary by several pounds and kilos depending on hundreds of different factors. Being a bit dehydrated like you are each morning or on a hot day can affect your weight by many pounds too.

The way to help with all of this statistical noise is to take lots and lots of readings. Write them all down and use a spreadsheet to plot a nice average plot line.

If you aren't able to do this many times a day then once a day at the same time will be ok. Don't forget that scales are not even a tiny bit accurate unless they are on a hard surface. Not on carpet. And if you can't work a spreadsheet, paper will be just dandy.

The point of measuring is once again using the Hawthorne effect. This psychological trick will help you lose weight by keeping you on task and your mind focused in the right direct. Each day. It really works. Do it.

twenty one
enjoy food

This is what I want you to try with food. Really savor it. Have nice food. Cook it well and enjoy each mouthful. Enjoy the look of it on the plate, notice the noises and sensation as it passes your lips. Smell it on the way in. Allow the aroma on the mouth-approach to herald the feel on your tongue and textures as your teeth go to work on it.

If you take time to enjoy your food rather than going piraña and trying to inhale it, you will probably appreciate it a lot more. Eating slowly is good for you. You will get less indigestion. You tend to shovel food in quickly if you don't concentrate. This leads to overeating. A painfully tight belly after a meal is not a good habit if you want a better waistline. Eating more slowly will enable you to taste your food better. If you enjoy your food you will appreciate it more.

Food is vital to stay alive, but eating too much of it makes us fat. We will, if left unchecked eat ourselves into an early grave. Each munchy mouthful nibbling and gnawing away at our life expectancy.

A way around this is to pay more attention to what we eat. Paying more attention allows us to notice more details. If we notice more details this can help us to eat in a more healthy manner.

Food comes with an array of different stuff to bombard all our senses and make the experience more sensual and enjoyable.

Colorful food attractively presented gets our salivary juices flowing. We anticipate what is coming next. Even before we see it, we can build anticipation using only our imagination (we can even slaver from simply reading a menu description or by fondly recalling some nice food we once ate). We hear the food at it arrives, as we cut it, bite it, chew it and crunch.

Our noses overhang our mouths. The nose gets a blast of what is coming. We inhale the scent particles and the smell of the food lends massively to its flavor.

Actually more than 90% of the taste of food comes from the smell part. Think of the last time you had a blocked nose or common cold and how bland food tasted. This is because our tongue can manage to distinguish and discern only a few separate tastes (bitter, sour, sweet, salt and umami - *umami is a sort of savory taste*). Everything else we taste with all of its complex and beautiful notes comes from the nose inhaled part. We have smell detectors right up at the top of the nose and these stick out of the very brain itself.

Take time to smell and appreciate food on the way in. You will find out lots and lots about what you are about to eat. Most people find that if you take time to enjoy the smell of food that the enjoyment levels go up much more than they imagined.

Imagination, sight, sound, smell, taste and touch. These are the six senses. Touching and feeling food is an important part of the eating experience. Not just with our fingers... Our lips and tongue are covered in touch sensors and we can detect tiny differences in texture, feel, grittiness, smoothness, mouth-feel and more. All of our body orifices are super-sensitive and if touched in the right way can feel quite nice. The mouth is included in these. This is the way we are made. Right out of the box. Use it. Enjoy and experience the way food feels on the way in. Enjoy it in your mouth, on your tongue, move it around and notice what it feels like on its way past your tongue and down the upper part of your throat as you swallow. The back of the tongue also has taste sensors, as does the upper part of the throat (*oropharynx*), if you give yourself a chance to notice what these tell you, the fore-tastes and after-tastes of food can be appreciated too.

Make nice food. Put nice food in. Eat well, you body will appreciate it. This encourages you to find more nutritious food to fuel your fabulous body. You will also eat more slowly and put less in. All good.

twenty two
eat slowly

You and I could go for a walk in the countryside. We might probably enjoy being outdoors and the sights, sounds and smells on the open trail. But if you *really* want to enjoy a walk like this you should **saunter**. I love the word saunter. Nobody knows where this word meaning to **wander slowly** comes from. Possibly from *santren*, meaning 'to muse' in Old English. A made up but more cuddly explanation comes from *à la Saint[e] Terre*, talking about pilgrims journeying to the Holy Land. This comes from the French words *Saint* and *terre*. This means walking as if you are on holy earth. I like to think this means you really take time to appreciate all the good stuff around, reverently treating the world you tread on with respect.

I know that sounds a little bit like woo woo and I promised this book would have no woo, but I think you will sense what I'm getting at. My grandmother, a housewife all her adult life used to say your tummy needed twenty minutes before it could tell you it was feeling full.

Twenty years of medicine later and I've learned nothing which says she was even a bit wrong. And much to back her up. The theory here is that if you can bring yourself to eat a little more slowly, you will then hear the full signal sooner and will therefore feel full and sated before you can shovel too many calories in that you really didn't need.

My Grandmother says eat slowly and you'll feel full faster.

Indeed true. As with trying to work out where the word saunter comes from, there are a few different plausible explanations. All probably partially correct. There are *stretch receptors* in the stomach. Put enough stuff in, they stretch and send nerve signals directly and chemical signals (*hormones* in the blood stream) indirectly back to your brain to tell you to slow down your eating as you are becoming fuller.

The same nerves and chemical signals are triggered by *chemo-receptors* embedded in the stomach wall. These detect food and its breakdown products and are able to signal to the brain to slow down eating.

These same and similar chemo-receptors are found in the top part of the small intestine (the *duodenum*) just after the outflow from the stomach. As the stomach empties past its muscular *pyloric sphincter*, these fire off to tell your brain that it can stop eating as it's got plenty to be processing.

This chain of events takes time. Not much, but enough that you can measure. The more careful and measured you are in the way that you eat stuff, the better these natural processes can signal to slow down the eating. They do this by decreasing your hunger level. Hunger is a rather non-specific feeling and is the sum of all these physical things and also your psychological brain stuff. Both equally important.

For the physical stuff, eating slowly and eating food with protein and fat will lead to you feeling fuller sooner. So much so that eating too much protein and fat triggers nausea. So you feel a bit sick. This will do the trick for encouraging you not to eat too much, but is probably best avoided. I want you to get a great waistline, but I don't want the process to be unpleasant. You want after all to be able to use the tips in this book for the rest of your life if you need to. You aren't going to listen to me or trust what I say if you feel unwell or unhappy about the whole thing.

twenty three
nothing which needs a label

Stuff with labels = bad.
Stuff without labels = good.

Ok, I know that's pretty simplistic, but it is a good rule of thumb.

Maybe extend the rule to stuff with packaging from a shop, versus stuff in a paper bag from a stall or farmers market. We are going to want to eat natural foods with lots of protein and fiber. Stuff with sugars and carbohydrates less so.

Stuff with labels and packaging includes; lasagna, chocolate, corn syrup, sodas, beer, ice cream, cookies, juice and cereals. Stuff with less packaging and fewer labels includes; tomatoes, nuts, eggs, vegetables, fruit, salad, cheese, milk, meat, chicken, fish, peas, beans and lentils.

Our digestive systems are 200,000 years old. As humans. Before that we go back several more millions of years. We are all beautifully constructed to get all of what we need from everything we can find and put in the top end. We evolved as hunter gatherers to eat a wide and varied diet of fish, meat, eggs, fruit, nuts, berries, roots and probably each other from time to time.

If you simply put in potatoes, bread and cookies you will not be doing yourself any favors. The sort of food which is better for you can nearly always be found without packaging or labels.

If it needs a label, consider avoiding it.

twenty five
would a caveman eat it?

We have the same biological set up on the inside of our bodies and brains to our ancestors of forty thousand years ago. When we all lived in East Africa in the Great Rift Valley our lives looked very different.

This was a long time before farming. We lived in small groups of up to one hundred and fifty people and would set up camp in an area for as long as there was picking, gathering and hunting to keep our bellies full. We then moved on. We were nomadic hunter-gatherers. Psychologically we needed the support and approval of our group and were distrustful of outsiders.

Food-wise we ate nuts, berries, fruit when we could get it and hunted occasionally. Small animals and birds were easier than big game. Not much milk, occasionally honey and probably few eggs. Certainly no domesticated livestock such as cows, pigs, goats, sheep or chickens. Our food we mostly ate raw. We hadn't got the hang of fire and cooking by that point.

Your biology is set up for the life of a nomadic caveman. If you eat this food, there is a good chance that you will be healthy and keep a decent weight.

There are conflicting opinions about just how good for you a paleolithic diet is. The *paleolithic* period of human history stretches from ten thousand years ago back for 2.5 million years. A long time. We did well as a species. We survived. Not only did we survive but we expanded to fill nearly every ecological niche on the entire planet (apart from underwater of course). And when we got there we pretty much killed off all significant predators and took over all the available landmass. Not bad for a fairly puny ape.

As with so many things in diet and nutrition, when you get past the hype the picture is actually a bit more complex. Caveman didn't eat much dairy, they didn't farm, there was no sugar and very few grains (ancient grains grew very poorly before we cultivated them). People claim that you will live longer, happier and healthier if you follow this. They usually claim that legumes too shouldn't be eaten (beans, peas, lentils). But ...

The picture is complex in that no convincing studies have been done to show this is at all helpful to follow. Humans excel at their adaptability, their guts included. We can eat and thrive on pretty much anything. So you probably don't need to exclude things from your diet like the fanatics would have us believe. A sensible way forward is to avoid high calorie processed foods. You *can* have grains but not too many. You can have legumes as part of a **balanced** diet. Having a **variety** of stuff is the key. Dairy doesn't need to be banned, it just shouldn't feature too heavily. The same with potatoes and bread.

Have plenty of protein, eat only natural fats and cut right back on carbohydrates. This is the **paleolithic approach**. Have lots of variety and eat plenty of fresh stuff. We can never prove what our ancestors ate and if they were any healthier or thinner than us. But these steps do make a lot of sense.

Interestingly this approach lends itself towards exclusion diets. Towards being dairy-free, alcohol-free, sugar-free, GM-free, organic, gluten-free and low-carbohydrate. These are popular diets that many people swear by. I feel they are perhaps too extreme as we evolved to cope with most stuff. But if we are trying to reverse the excesses of our waistline energy storage, the *paleo* approach seems to have a lot going for it.

Don't forget that we didn't cook much food either. All of this adds up to a lot of food that was much harder to digest than modern food. Stuff that needed a lot more chewing and had an awful lot more fiber. You will do well to have lots and lots of fiber in your food.

The variety of foods we eat these days (I sound like my grandparents now) is very small, we should broaden it. When we do this we will find it easier to get all the vitamins and minerals we need. We will find it easier not to overeat.

If in doubt:

Ask yourself, would a caveman eat this?

If the answer is no, then don't eat that. If you are a healthy, happy weight, then do what you like. Up until that point keep asking yourself the question. It will help you.

twenty six
don't eat to fill an emotional hole

We are designed to enjoy food. If we don't eat, we die. To encourage our ancestors to eat rather than just procreate and sleep, hunger evolved. Along with the feel-good sensation of a full belly.

We are designed to get a bit of pleasure each time we fill our belly. A bit of comfort with eating and with eating to being pretty full. Nearly to bursting. Painfully full isn't just painful, it sort of feels a bit nice. That used to be a survival advantage. But it can now be our undoing.

Many of us aren't happy all the time. Lots of us have a bit of a rough deal and can't do much about it. When life feels a bit rubbish, we sometimes fill our bellies to give ourselves a bit of a comfort feeling. This works (*a bit*), otherwise we wouldn't do it. But it only works for a few minutes. Then the sad feelings remain. Sometimes remorse follows and regret about having just eaten our own bodyweight in unnecessary snacks. We can then feel even worse.

Comfort eating: understandable, but pretty unhelpful.

It is important to try and spot when it is happening and see if there are some better ways you can go about getting some comfort, reassurance, validation, emotional support or simple distraction from whichever problems are plaguing you that day. Look for some other ways around these obstacles and try not to hoover the calories.

There are some tell-tale ways to spot whether you are *properly hungry* or about to eat to fill an *emotional* hole. If you are **properly hungry**, this comes on slowly and will fade after a while before coming back to remind you. Like an alarm clock on snooze. This is simply your body reminding you that you need to eat. The animal unconscious part of your brain reminding the human part in case it has forgotten.

Emotional hunger tends to come on at a rush and it can feel more urgent. It is your animal brain giving you an emotion and your human brain interprets this incorrectly. It can seem overwhelming. If that is that case, eating won't make it go away for more than a few minutes. Learning to recognize it and finding better ways of making the emotion go away will be better for your waistline. It will be better for your emotional wellbeing too.

Emotional hunger doesn't make your tummy growl. That is real hunger. Having a tummy rumble and hearing the *borborygmi* is an excellent way to tell you it is time to eat. If you don't feel or hear this, you can safely put-off and delay your eating.

If you feel guilt, shame, regret or remorse after you have eaten, you were probably not really hungry. If you are eating to fuel your body, that is something to be pleased about. If you feel bad afterwards, have a think about why that might be. This is a clue you may have been eating to fill an emotional hole.

If you are in need of a bit more love, comfort, human connection or are feeling tired or stressed, please don't eat to make this go away. It will help only briefly and will not make the original problem go away. Try keeping an emotional diary of your thoughts or feelings. This can help with controlling your emotions.

- If you are anxious, try finding a distracting activity until the wave passes.

- If you are tired - sleep is the answer, not food.

- If you are stressed, you either need to get more help or move the goalposts in such a way that it no longer bothers you as much. Again, snacks are not a great way of dealing with stress and pressure.

twenty seven
set artificial rules

- **600 cal days**
- **eight to eight**
- **nothing white**
- **nothing in the car**

Rules. Do you like them?

I don't either. Some people reckon that rules are there to be followed by people not smart enough to view them as guidelines. But I digress.

Some of my patients find that they are able to make more rapid progress if they give themselves artificial rules. They make up a rule and then behave as if there was a proper reason for following it. Like it was some kind of law or something and the police or FBI would find out and come after you if you broke it.

These can be really useful. Because you get to make up rules that benefit you. One favorite is having some days when you can *only have 600 calories*. That's it. No more. When you get to your maximum, you have to go hungry. Clearly you can do what you like and can reach for the candy bars when you hit 600, so the situation is artificial. But having the rule that you follow on certain days is a good way of marshaling what goes in. Some people find the psychological constraint of the rule is in some ways easier to follow than trying to restrict a bit what goes in. This is the logic behind intermittent fasting. Like the popular five-two diet (fast on two days a week, eat normally on the rest).

Having no food in the car is a great rule.

Also *have no snacks visible* in the kitchen or within arms reach of anywhere comfortable, like your sofa.

Don't allow yourself to eat after eight in the evening. This is used by many people as the 8:8 diet. *Nothing after eight in the evening and nothing before eight in the morning.* Every day of the week regardless of what you are doing. It is easy to remember, works quite well and teaches self-discipline. It has the added bonus of decreasing your options to snack when you are tired. Definitely worth a try if you're looking for ideas. Most people find this one quite easy, do-able from day one and it can be safely done indefinitely.

Try riding the wave when hunger strikes. Surf it baby!

If you are hungry, hit the mental snooze alarm:

- Wait five to ten minutes and see if you are just as hungry.
- Walk around the block.
- Go and tidy the kitchen.
- Vacuum the car.
- Distract yourself for a short while.

If you are still hungry, then go and eat. If not, give yourself a pat on the back and congratulate yourself. This sounds silly to some of my patients but is an important step. When you get something right when you do something helpful, reward this. Like training a puppy. Reward the good stuff. You will naturally want to do more of it.

twenty eight
no bored snacking

When we aren't entertained we become bored.

We are designed to be mentally busy a lot of the time. Busy gathering food, eating food, finding, attracting and then having sex with potential mates. Busy rearing and looking after children, nursing our aging relatives and so on.

Modern society has made us a lot more efficient at all of those. That frees up spare time. In the spare time, the brain wanders aimlessly. It doesn't just switch off, but it will do stuff without aim or direction unless you point it somewhere. And you may end up snacking without really noticing.

As humans we don't like to be overwhelmed. We like to be whelmed. That is where everything is just right. The **Goldilocks zone** (not too hot, not too cold, but just right).

If you are underwhelmed, you will be bored. If you are bored, one of the things you may well do is gorge on calorie laden snacks. This will make you more porcine and not be helpful in your quest for a beach-ready body. Notice when you are bored and either hide the snacks or go and entertain yourself in a productive manner.

Noticing when you do this is the first part of the process. If you suspect this could apply to you, using a food diary is one of your best ways to address this. Write down everything you put in your mouth each day. Drinks included. Many calories can be consumed in liquid form. Often without noticing. If it contains ice cream like a shake then that is obvious. Fruit juices are just as bad and many of my patients falsely assume they are healthy because the packaging looks friendly. Don't trust the packaging.

Flavored water is packaged nicely but comes loaded with sugar. Be cautious, careful and write it all down. The Hawthorne effect of focused attention will help your waistline project too.

__Beware of liquid calories. They are sneaky, my precious.__

When you write everything down, you may start to see patterns emerge of when you eat because you are bored. If you spot this, find other stuff to do. Get a plan. Ask your weight loss buddy what they do if you need inspiration. Look on the line to see what other people do if you get really stuck.

twenty nine
no distracted eating

When I was growing up I sometimes went to the cinema for a treat. Birthdays and so on. When we were there we would forever be pestering to have popcorn. Popcorn and films used to go hand-in-hand. Some of us have extended those childhood habits to involve watching anything.

When we sit down to watch TV, a sports game, a film, gameshow or even a chat show, many of us reach for the snacks. And we usually aren't selecting the healthiest options.

When we are distracted we can absentmindedly eat an awful lot of calories. We can do this on the sofa, in the car and even in bed.

The cure is in becoming more aware of what is going in. This means not concentrating wholly on whatever the distraction and instead focusing on the hand coming towards our mouth. I do know this is usually less interesting. But you need to stop the automatic behaviour. Dead in its tracks. Stop the hand movements. We need a rule to follow:

No food to be allowed in when you aren't fully aware.

Make it your rule. An artificial rule, I grant you. You get to make and break these whenever you like. But this is a good one. You can of course eat when you like. You are a grown up and you get to make your grown up choices on your own. But only eating when you are going to enjoy it, savor it and notice what is going in will help you with your quest and keep you on track to achieve your target. You know it makes sense.

Being busy is a great way to lose weight.

I mean really busy. Running away from tigers, running for a bus, last-minute Christmas shopping, cleaning the kitchen before the in-laws arrive. These and many other things in our day-to-day lives keep us busy.

When we are super-busy, occasionally we forget to eat. We can even miss meals sometimes. This is because our brains are wired to be able to do stuff to live, thrive and survive. We can last on our fuel tanks for a very long time if we have to. Because you can last for ages, this means you don't always have to be eating to survive. That would be grazing and you are not a cow or horse. Remember that.

thirty
no procrastinating by eating

When you've got stuff to do that you know you really *should* do, you probably won't want to do it.

Most of us put stuff off. This is normal. It is part of the human condition.

In fact, if you always do whatever needs to be done and don't have a cluttered inbox and piles of paper everywhere, unpaid bills and even unopened ones, this marks you out as being more weird than if you do, it's that common. Just because a lot of people do it, that doesn't make it a good idea. Just think of the proverbial lemming. But that is for another book (***Do it, do it, DO IT!*** - *A Procrastinator's Guide to World Domination*, in case you were wondering. Whenever I get around to writing it).

Some people watch TV to procrastinate. Some people read the paper, some surf the web. If you are looking at *LOLcats* or watching funny animal videos, you are probably putting something off. Some people go out drinking beer, some stay in. Some people indulge in quiet me-time. The rest of us eat. We overeat. We shovel the snacks in and do anything other than what we should be doing.

This is doubly bad. Nothing gets done and we get bigger. Our middles expand and we still have stuff to do. Disaster. One cure:

Stop eating (or whatever else you were doing) and get on with it.

Or buy my other book. Anything you like, but stop eating when you should be doing other stuff. It is not helpful and you will probably regret it. Nuff said.

- Just do it.
- Crack on with it.
- No pussyfooting around.
- Action today.
- Don't be munching to put it off.

- Don't be buying food, preparing food, cooking food or eating food.
- You need **action, yes.**
- **Foody actions**, no.

There are two main ways to get yourself into action and out of procrastination mode: *Softly softly* and *massive kick up the rear end.*

Softly softly involves doing things so tiny and small that your brain can't object. If you are writing a book and struggling to make progress, you could set yourself a daily target of one sentence. It doesn't even have to be a good sentence. You can always edit it later.

Simply get it down on paper. Each day. Every day. And the next. And so on. Give yourself permission to write more if you want. As the days go by, the book will slowly start to take shape. And there it is. You've started.

The other method of beating procrastination is to take on a task *so* huge you can't think of how you can manage it. If you want to get fit, don't just go for a run. Enter a marathon! You will then need to take massive action. You can't ignore your goal. You will have to get off your butt every day if you are going to shift your bulk around a marathon of 26.2 miles come race day. You will need to cut your TV watching and get out for runs. You will need to cancel your regular cake order. You will need to skip some breakfasts. You will need to drink water not beer every night. And so on.

This is such a big undertaking that it can't just be put off. Because you need to act and you need something each and every day before the race comes. You can have a few off days. But not many.

This is a **massive kick up the rear end**. And into action. Take on something so massive that the only way to achieve it is to completely rearrange your life to be able to fit it in.

I don't care how you get over procrastination as long as it is productive and you are not eating and munching your way through calories while putting off the actions you know you really *should* be taking. I can't do it for you. This is your thing...

Go on then: Make a start.

I'll wait.

thirty one
no sad snacks, no comfort binges

I know the cover says thirty. But this is important:

I know we've sort of covered snacking when you should be doing something else. And we've covered not filling you face when you should be; having a hug, calling your mum, making up with your partner, going for a run, writing poetry, playing an instrument, reading a novel, writing your novel, doing your tax returns or whatever else you need to be doing to make your heart and your brain happier. But...

This is important and so many of my patients come unstuck on this, I'm going to labor the point.

Do not try to fill an emotional hole with food. It will plug the gap. But *only temporarily*. This transient relief will vanish and leave you feeling hollow. Notice what you are about to do. Stop. Give yourself a big pat on the back for noticing and go and do something else. Distract yourself. Find a way to make yourself feel better which doesn't involve empty calories.

It can involve food, but prepare yourself something nourishing. Something with protein, fiber and healthy, natural ingredients. Then eat it slowly and enjoy the flavors.

No sad snacks.

If you eat to feel better, the relief will be transient at best. The feelings fade but the calories last. It's really easy to do and a hard habit to break. If you can catch yourself and stop yourself in the act, you can start the first step in making this habit a thing of the past.

When you notice it happening, reward yourself. Not with cake, but a non-calorific gold star. You may well find yourself reaching for calories when it is emotional hunger several times a day at first. Do something different. You will know in your life what that could be.

Send an email, text or tweet. Check in with friends or relatives, even on the book of faces or by *Skype*. Go for a walk, tidy your bedroom, clean the kitchen. Do something. Anything. But most of all, when you are feeling sad and lonely, go easy on the food intake. It's just not going to be the best thing for you right now.

Plan: *chin up and change direction.*

and finally…
when you fall off that wagon

Let us face it. It will happen. Plan for this.

Having an off day, a moment of weakness, a special occasion, the social pressure of a wedding, a partner's birthday and so on. The excuses are endless and the occasions limitless.

It's gonna happen. To you.

That's ok, you are human. The trick is not to make it every day. Or even every other day. Preferably not even once a week. All the extra you eat on the off days will go somewhere. That will need reversing.

Don't beat yourself up though. To be human is, err, only human. And as a human you will screw stuff up. Well, maybe you are better than me and only mess up a couple of times a month, but I screw stuff up. A lot. Most days I find stuff I could have done better. Should have done better. Knew better than to do and say what I did.

But I'm working on it. I try to keep those down to a minimum, and I usually don't let on. Lots of them pass by unnoticed by others. Or, at least they don't tell me to my face. I'm not sure whether that is a good thing or a bad thing. But the point is, I mess up and so do most people. When we try harder stuff, we increase the chances that it won't go completely to plan.

Dieting, managing our waistline, shaping our beach-ready bodies is going to be a little tougher as each year passes. Whatever your current state and your goal, it is a fairly good bet that you will have to put in a bit of effort. It is also a good bet that things will not go perfectly each and every day.

That is ok. It's the same for all of us. It is in what you do about the wrinkles, the bumps in the road and the rocks to climb over. This is where the magic lies:

- Think of the rocks as stepping stones and look at the bigger picture.
- Don't get hung up on each trip or stumble.
- Chin up.
- Dry those tears.
- Dust yourself off.
- Fix on the horizon, look at your goal.
- Keep your eyes on the prize and get your feet moving.

That's the way.

bonus
BetterNights

People who sleep better lose weight faster and more easily. But many people struggle with their sleep. They feel stressed, have weight problems and low energy levels. Following these rules can help. A lot. These rules have medical science to back them. Don't take my word for it. Try them out. Today.

Follow these for a fortnight. If you are no worse, then do another fortnight and make it the month.

The sleep rules:

1. **Get a bed time routine**. Teeth, pajamas, set alarm, write in journal. That sort of thing.
2. **Stop mental stimulation before bed**. No electronic gadgets or TV in the bedroom is a good rule. Reading is ok. No texting / sexting or emails if you are struggling.
3. **Have a dark sleeping place**. Consider black-out blinds / eye mask.
4. **Have a quiet sleeping place**. If noise bothers you, wear earplugs.
5. **Have a safe feeling sleeping place**. Consider an intruder alarm and install extra locks.
6. **Avoid anything with blue light** (TV, computer, smartphone, tablet) **for three hours before bed**. If you really must, use amber sunglasses to cut this unhelpful light (you may look silly but will thank me for the tip). Reading books is ideal (*Kindle* / *Kobo* are ok).
7. **Don't eat before bed**. You don't need it, and will sleep anyway even if a little peckish.
8. **Don't drink after your evening meal**. Full bladders help no one.
9. **Cut alcohol**. To zero. Alcohol keeps your bladder active at night (**bad**), overhydrates you (**bad**) and will sedate you which stops effective dreaming (**bad**).
10. **Cut all caffeine after lunchtime** if you are sleeping ok and remove all caffeine for a fortnight if you are struggling. Note: *Green tea and many body building / herbal supplements contain caffeine.*

Keep a sleep diary. Write four entries each night:

- Two on retiring (worry list, grateful list).
- Two on rising (how well you slept and your dream recollections).
- Write your stresses on a piece of paper before bed. Your sleeping brain will help sort through these during the night.
- Write a grateful list - three things you are grateful for (this is proven to lift mood).

Plan your dreams. They can be shaped by pre-planning nice stuff to dream about (or a thorny problem to work through). As you fall asleep allow your mind to wander. Give yourself permission to sift through any worries knowing you will process them while you slumber.

As you drift off, float to a beautiful fantasy land (nothing too stimulating). Furnish it to taste, make it warm, comfortable, beautiful scenes, calming and tranquil. My favorite is to be safely stretched out in the sunshine at a fabulous lakeside cabin with mountain views.

Get some fresh air each morning. Outside bright morning light helps set your body clock.

Allow naps. Three o'clock in the afternoon works well for most:

- **Short** 1-15 minute naps boost energy levels.
- **Medium** 20-40 minute naps decrease stress levels.
- **Longer** 45-90 minute naps improve productivity and give a huge recharge boost to your day.

Go to bed early but try to rise at the same time each day. Most of us get nowhere near the 8+ hours we need each night. You cannot bank sleep and you cannot catch up properly in a weekend.

Review your progress at the end of the month. If you're still struggling, consult your doctor.

about the author

Thank you for reading my book. If you enjoyed it, please leave a review online.

———

Dr Phil Harley enjoys running. And some other stuff. Mostly running. He lives in the New Forest, UK.

If you have any comments, thoughts, questions or feedback, please email drphil@brainsolutions.co.uk

———

More information at www.brainsolutions.co.uk
Other books by Dr Harley:

Out now

Skinny Genes - *Weight Gain Explained & the CURE*

Desert Marathon Training - *2nd edition: Tips for Beginners*

Beginner's Guide to Running

Ultramarathon Running Injuries - *Niggles, scrapes and nipple chafes*

Doctor Secrets for Easy Weight Loss - *Ten simple steps for success; Real weight loss, for real people in the real world, which really works.*

Coming soon

Stand Up Sexy - *Perfect Posture for Everyday & Better Bedroom Fun*

Do it, Do it, *DO IT!* - *A Procrastinator's Guide to World Domination*

Stand Up Sexy - *Perfect Posture for Everyday & Better Bedroom Fun. Cure Back Pain - A Doctor's Guide*